Hair Structure and Chemistry Simplified

WORKBOOK

Fifth Edition

JOHN HALAL

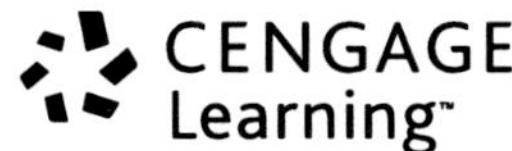

Australia • Brazil • Japan • Korea • Mexico • Singapore • Spain • United Kingdom • United States

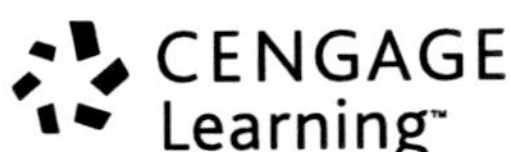

Hair Structure and Chemistry Simplified Workbook, Fifth Edition
John Halal

President, Milady: Dawn Gerrain

Publisher: Erin O'Connor

Acquisitions Editor: Martine Edwards

Product Manager: Jessica Burns

Editorial Assistant: Mike Spring

Director of Beauty Industry Relations: Sandra Bruce

Marketing Manager: Gerard McAvey

Production Director: Wendy Troeger

Senior Content Project Manager: Nina Tucciarelli

Art Director: Joy Kocsis

Technology Project Manager: Sandy Charette

Library of Congress Control Number: 2007941007

ISBN-13: 978-1-4283-3561-5

ISBN-10: 1-4283-3561-7

Milady
Executive Woods
5 Maxwell Drive
Clifton Park, NY 12065
USA

Cengage Learning is a leading provider of customized learning solutions with office locations around the globe, including Singapore, the United Kingdom, Australia, Mexico, Brazil, and Japan. Locate your local office at **www.cengage.com/global**

Cengage Learning products are represented in Canada by Nelson Education, Ltd.

To learn more about Milady, visit **milady.cengage.com**

Purchase any of our products at your local college store or at our preferred online store **www.cengagebrain.com**

Printed in the United States of America
3 4 5 6 7 22 21 20 19 18

Contents

How to Use This Workbook

Milady's *Workbook to Accompany Hair Structure and Chemistry Simplified, Fifth Edition,* has been written to accompany Milady's textbook, *Hair Structure and Chemistry Simplified, Fifth Edition.* This book directly follows the information found in that book.

Students are to answer each item in this workbook after reading/studying their textbook for correct information. Items can be corrected and/or rated during class or individual discussions, or on an independent study basis.

At the end of each chapter is a word review. Students are encouraged to write down the definitions of these key words. They may also be used as study guides, for class discussions, or for the instructor to assign groups of words to individual students or groups of students to define.

At the end of the book is a review test, which is an evaluation of all 15 chapters in the book. There are 150 items on this test—10 items from each chapter in numerical order. This may be given as one large test, or divided into 15 small tests.

John Halal

Date ____________________

Rating ____________________

Text Pages 1–8

Chapter 1 Science and Cosmetology

WHAT IS SCIENCE?

1. Define *science*.

____

2. Science is a logical system which helps us to learn more about what we do not ____________________.

3. List three basic steps of the scientific system for learning.

   1. ____

   2. ____

   3. ____

4. A. Identify two parts of our body that are used for observation.

   1. ____

   2. ____

   B. List three observations that can be used in cosmetology.

   1. ____

   2. ____

   3. ____

5. A. Define power of *reasoning*.

____

   B. Reasoning turns ____________________ into useful ideas.

   C. Identify the basis of faulty reasoning.

____

6. A. What is the best way to test ideas and knowledge?

____

B. Testing ideas allows a person to:

1. ____

2. ____

C. Identify one way to test new cosmetology products.

____

D. List two items on which good experiments are based.

1. ____

2. ____

7. A very important area of study for scientists is ____________________ something happens. Scientists study the ____________________ of an event.

8. A. Whose instructions should you follow when using any product or chemical?

____

B. Define incompatible mixtures.

____

C. List five possible reactions of incompatible mixtures.

1. ____

2. ____

3. ____

4. ____

5. ____

D. Identify two common cleansers that can be deadly when mixed together.

1. ______________________________

2. ______________________________

9. Claims such as "miracle skin cream" and "revolutionary new product" are advertising and

______________ tools and are not true ______________.

WORD REVIEW

ammonia
cause and effect
chlorine bleach
experimenting
faulty reasoning
incompatible mixtures
manufacturer's instructions
miracle
observation
poor observations
power of reasoning
reasoning
science

Date ______________________

Rating ______________________

Text Pages 9–16

Chapter 2 The Structure of Life

1. Define *biology*.

____

2. A. The "backbone of nature" is ____________________.

   B. List three items that are made with "the backbone of nature."

   1. ____

   2. ____

   3. ____

3. A. After each letter below, identify the correct element name.

   1. C stands for ____________________

   2. H stands for ____________________

   3. O stands for ____________________

   4. N stands for ____________________

   5. S stands for ____________________

   B. The five elements in Question 3.A make up what percent of the body?

   ____

   C. List three cosmetology-related areas of the body made by the COHNS elements.

   1. ____

   2. ____

   3. ____

4. Matching: Match the terms on the left with their correct descriptions on the right.

______________ 1. molecules	A. there are 77 of these found in nature
______________ 2. organic compounds	B. these are formed when atoms of different elements combine with each other
______________ 3. compound molecules	C. anything that is, or ever was, alive
______________ 4. cells	D. the control center of a cell
______________ 5. elements	E. compounds that contain carbon
______________ 6. organic	F. there are about 90 of these found in nature
	G. the technical name for cell division
	H. these are formed when atoms combine with each other
	I. microscopic communities of millions of large molecules grouped together

5. A. Define *organic*.

____

B. List eight items that are "organic."

1. ____
2. ____
3. ____
4. ____
5. ____
6. ____
7. ____
8. ____

C. Are "organic" products better, healthier, safer, or more natural than other products?

Check one:

_______ yes

_______ no

CELLS

6. The word *cell* comes from a Latin word for ________________________.

7. How many cells are in your body?

____

8. How fast do cells die and replace themselves?

____

9. List five cell functions/purposes.

1. ____
2. ____
3. ____
4. ____
5. ____

10. Identify the parts of a cell in the illustration below.

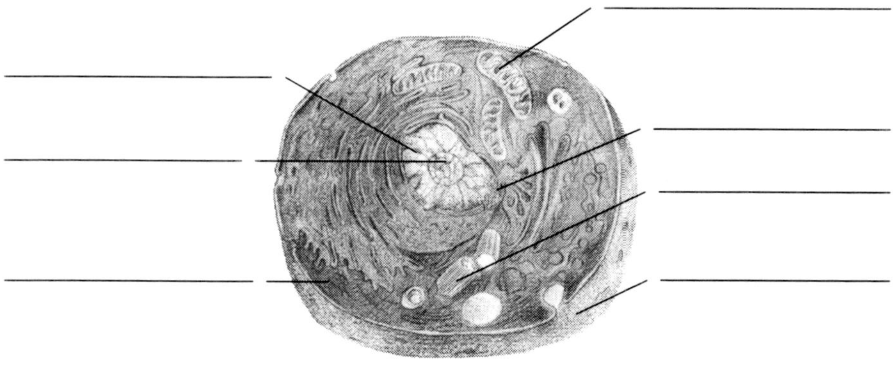

11. Identification Match: Match the characteristics listed below with the correct parts of a cell.

cell membrane/wall
nucleus
cytoplasm

Characteristics:

_______________ 1. directs activity and organizes its work

_______________ 2. a clear, jelly-like substance

_______________ 3. the control center

_______________ 4. separates it from other cells

_______________ 5. small bodies float in this

_______________ 6. allows food in and passes waste out

12. A. Define *organelle*.

____

B. One organelle, which is called the "powerhouse" of the cell because it supplies the cell its energy, is the

_______________.

13. A. Identify three reasons why cells die quickly.

1. ____

2. ____

3. ____

B. Cells reproduce as the nucleus stretches and splits in _______________.

C. What is the name for this process of cell division?

____

14. A. What is entropy?

____

B. What is the natural state of matter?

____

C. What is the "Miracle of Life"?

____

15. A. Explain the process of keratinization.

____

____

B. How long does it take for the epidermis to completely renew itself?

____

C. How long does it take for a new cell to reach the stratum corneum?

____

16. A. Groups of cells combine to make ______________________.

B. Groups of tissues combine to make ______________________.

C. Groups of organs combine to make ______________________.

WORD REVIEW

biology
building blocks
carbon
cell membrane/wall
cells
COHNS
compounds
cytoplasm
elements
mitochondria
mitosis
molecules
nucleus
organelles
organic
organic molecules
organs
systems
tissues

Date ______________

Rating ______________

Text Pages 17–24

Chapter 3 Microbiology

INTRODUCTION

1. A. List two other names for microorganisms.

   1. ______________
   2. ______________

   B. Why is it important to understand how microorganisms grow and spread?

   ____

   ____

   C. What are bacteria?

   ____

   D. What is bacteriology?

   ____

BACTERIA

2. A. What is the difference between pathogenic bacteria and nonpathogenic bacteria?

   ____

   ____

   B. List six benefits of nonpathogenic bacteria.

   1. ______________
   2. ______________
   3. ______________
   4. ______________

5. ____________________

6. ____________________

C. What are saprophytes?

____

D. What are the two most common types of pathogens?

1. ____________________

2. ____________________

E. List the three main classes of pathogenic bacteria and indicate their distinctive shapes.

1. ____________________

2. ____________________

3. ____________________

F. What are motile bacteria?

____

G. List two types of motile bacteria.

1. ____________________

2. ____________________

H. What are the names of the two different structures that bacteria use to propel themselves through liquids?

1. ____________________

2. ____________________

BACTERIAL GROWTH AND REPRODUCTION

3. A. What are the two distinct stages in the life cycle of bacteria?

1. ____________________

2. ____________________

B. Why is the inactive stage of special concern in cosmetology?

____

C. List four ways that viruses are different from bacteria.

1. ______________________________

2. ______________________________

3. ______________________________

4. ______________________________

D. What do the letters AIDS stand for?

____

E. What is the virus that causes AIDS?

____

F. List and define four infectious agents other than bacteria and viruses.

1. ______________________________

2. ______________________________

3. ______________________________

4. ______________________________

G. What is the difference between a local and a general infection?

____

____

H. List the two types of immunity.

1. ______________________________

2. ______________________________

Date ______________________

Rating ______________________

Text Pages 25–42

Chapter 4 The Structure of Skin

TISSUE

1. Define *tissue*.

____

2. Identification Match: Using the terms listed below, match the characteristics with the correct tissue type.

connective tissue
muscular tissue
nerve tissue
liquid tissue
epithelial tissue

Characteristics:

______________________ 1. carries food to cells and removes waste

______________________ 2. gives a protective covering to the body

______________________ 3. examples are cartilage, ligaments, and tendons

______________________ 4. sends messages to the brain

______________________ 5. when they contract or relax, movement occurs

______________________ 6. examples are the linings of the stomach, heart, and lungs

______________________ 7. supports and protects the organs

______________________ 8. examples are blood and lymph

______________________ 9. gives the ability to move

______________________ 10. carries instructions from the brain to other body parts

3. Explain cell "specialization."

____

SKIN

4. What is skin?

____

5. List three harmful items to which skin is a barrier.

   1. _______________
   2. _______________
   3. _______________

6. A. How big is the skin?

   ____

   B. The skin weighs _______________ pounds.

7. A. Identify six items found in the subcutaneous tissue.

   1. _______________
   2. _______________
   3. _______________
   4. _______________
   5. _______________
   6. _______________

   B. Another name for adipose tissue is _______________.

   C. Identify four purposes/functions of adipose tissue.

   1. _______________
   2. _______________
   3. _______________
   4. _______________

8. A. Identify the percentage of the skin's dry weight that is made up by the dermis.

____

B. Identify the name of the lower part of the dermis.

____

C. Collagen is a substance used to make ______________ and makes up 75% of the skin's ______________. Its purpose is to give the skin strength and ______________.

D. Elastin gives skin the ability to ______________ and yet keep its shape. It accounts for only ______________% of the skin's dry weight. As skin ages, it contains ______________ elastin, and it becomes less ______________.

9. A. When do "mast cells" perform their function/s?

____

B. Mast cells first release a chemical that stops ______________. Later, they increase the flow of ______________ to the injury.

10. A. Identify two purposes/functions of the cells of the epidermis.

1. ____

2. ____

B. How thick is the epidermis?

____

C. Compare the size of the epidermis with that of the dermis.

____

D. How many layers are found within the epidermis?

____

E. Identify another name for "layer."

F. How long does it take for a new cell to reach the stratum corneum?

G. What size particles can pass through the skin and into the bloodstream?

11. Identification Match: Using the terms listed below, match the characteristics with the correct layer of the skin.

stratum germinativum
stratum granulosum
stratum lucidum
stratum corneum

Characteristics:

______________________ 1. the barrier that repels bacteria and light

______________________ 2. the cells begin to die here

______________________ 3. mitosis occurs here

______________________ 4. the cells no longer contain a nucleus

______________________ 5. the barrier that repels some chemicals

______________________ 6. the first step in keratin formation

______________________ 7. this layer is about 30 rows thick

______________________ 8. the basement of the epidermis

______________________ 9. transparent to light

______________________ 10. the beginning point of an upward journey

12. Identify and insert the names of the parts of the skin missing from the illustration below.

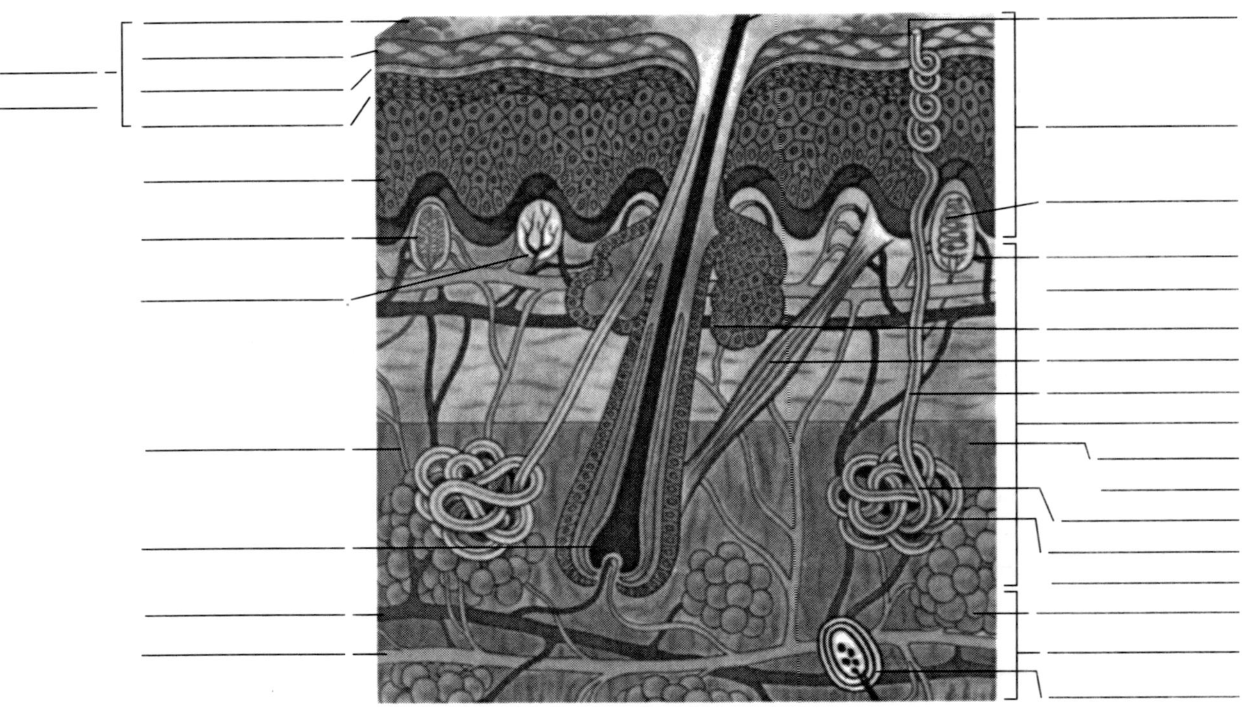

13. A. Explain the purpose of nerve endings.

____

B. Identify the number of nerve endings that are found in the skin.

____

14. Identification Match: Using the terms listed below, match the characteristics with the correct type of nerve.

sensory nerves
secretory nerves
motor nerves

Characteristics:

______________________ 1. cause gooseflesh/goosebumps

______________________ 2. send warning messages to prevent harm

______________________ 3. control the sebaceous glands

______________________ 4. pick up sensations

______________________ 5. make the hair shaft stand on end

______________________ 6. touch, pressure, heat, and cold

______________________ 7. control the sweat glands

15. A. Another name for the sweat gland is the ______________________ gland.

    B. Explain the sweat gland's purpose.

    ____

    C. Sweat reaches the skin through the ______________________.

16. A. Another name for sebaceous gland is ______________________ gland.

    B. Identify two parts of the body that do NOT contain sebaceous glands.

    1. ____

    2. ____

    C. How many sebaceous glands are on the scalp?

    ____

    D. Identify three purposes of sebum.

    1. ____

    2. ____

    3. ____

17. A. What type of gland has ducts that lead from the gland to a particular part of the body?

    ____

B. List two examples of glands that have ducts.

1. ______________________________

2. ______________________________

18. A. What type of gland is ductless and secretes hormones directly into the bloodstream?

____

19. A. List three factors that determine skin color.

1. ______________________________

2. ______________________________

3. ______________________________

B. Explain how blushing occurs.

____

C. What is melanin?

____

D. A person whose hair and skin contain NO melanin is known as a/an ______________________.

E. Besides melanin, another pigment that affects skin color is ______________________.

20. A. 90% of all skin cancers are the result of exposure to ______________________.

B. Each blistering sunburn increases the chance of developing skin cancer by ______________________.

C. Sunlight is made up of varying wavelengths of ______________________.

D. List the three main divisions of ultraviolet radiation.

1. ______________________________

2. ______________________________

3. ______________________________

21. A. Which type of UV rays cause erythema and tanning?

____

B. These are the longest wavelengths of ultraviolet radiation.

____

C. These are the UV rays that have the most energy.

____

D. These are the UV rays that penetrate the deepest.

____

E. Which type of UV rays are often referred to as the burning rays?

____

F. Most of these rays are blocked by ozone in the atmosphere.

____

22. A. What do the letters SPF stand for?

____

B. An SPF of 30 provides how much more protection than an SPF of 15?

____

C. What is the maximum SPF rating allowed by the FDA?

____

23. According to the proposed FDA rating system for UVA sunscreen products, what is the degree of protection for the following ratings?

A. Four Stars

____

B. One Star

____

24. What three steps should you take for maximum sunscreen protection?

1. ____

2. ____

3. ____

WORD REVIEW

adipose/fat tissue
albino
carotene
collagen
connective tissue
dermis
elastin
electromagnetic radiation
endocrine
epidermis
epithelial tissue
erythema
exocrine
infrared rays
keratin
liquid tissue
mast cells
melanin
motor nerves
muscular tissue
natural moisturizing factor
nerve tissue
reticular layer
sebaceous/oil gland
sebum
secretory nerves
sensory nerves
skin specialization
squalene
stratum corneum
stratum germinativum
stratum granulosum
stratum lucidum
subcutaneous tissue
sudoriferous/sweat glands
sun protection factor/SPF
sweat duct
tissue
ultraviolet radiation
visible light

Date ______________________

Rating ______________________

Text Pages 43–54

Chapter 5 Understanding Skin Disease

WHY DO COSMETOLOGISTS HAVE SKIN PROBLEMS?

1. How common are skin diseases in the United States as an occupation-related disease?

____

2. List four body areas where skin disorders commonly occur on cosmetologists.

   1. ____
   2. ____
   3. ____
   4. ____

TYPES OF SKIN DISEASE

3. Explain the cause of irritant contact dermatitis.

____

4. Which two skin layers can be chemically damaged?

   1. ____
   2. ____

5. List five symptoms of irritant contact dermatitis.

   1. ____
   2. ____
   3. ____
   4. ____
   5. ____

6. A. Chemicals that cause immediate, acute, and sometimes irreversible skin damage are called

   ______________________.

   B. Who should give medical treatment for the type of injury in question 6A?

   ____

7. What causes dandruff?

   ____

8. Define allergic contact dermatitis.

   ____

9. How long does it take to become allergic to a product?

   ____

10. Define sensitization.

    ____

11. Another name for sensitizers is ______________________.

12. The more often you use sensitizing chemicals, the greater your risk of becoming

    ______________________.

13. List three ways in which allergic contact dermatitis is different from irritant contact dermatitis.

    1. ____

    2. ____

    3. ____

14. List two cosmetology products that commonly cause allergic contact dermatitis.

    1. ____

    2. ____

15. What triggers an allergic reaction?

____

____

16. List two possible results of a severe allergic reaction.

1. ____

2. ____

17. Are there people who are not allergic to poison ivy?

____

____

18. List five other common names for formaldehyde.

1. ____

2. ____

3. ____

4. ____

5. ____

INFECTIONS

19. What causes a skin infection?

____

____

20. What are the four groups of pathogens that cause infection?

1. ____

2. ____

3. ______________________________

4. ______________________________

21. What is the most common type of bacterial infection?

____

22. What is *tinea pedis?*

____

23. What causes scabies?

____

____

24. What is a virus?

____

25. Identify one of the most common metal allergens in the world.

____

GLOVES

26. Discuss the benefits of wearing gloves in a salon.

____

27. List six style choices of gloves.

1. ______________________________

2. ______________________________

3. ______________________________

4. ______________________________

5. ______________________________

6. ______________________________

28. Some people become allergic to gloves that are made of ________________________.

29. Identify each of the following diseases as contagious or not contagious.

Verruca/wart	________________
Impetigo communicable	________________
Tinea communicable	________________
Herpes simplex virus	________________
Pityriasis (dandruff)	________________
Tinea favosa scalp	________________
Tinea capitis	________________
Pityriasis steatoides	________________
Furuncle	________________
Carbuncle/boil	________________
Tinea versicolor/yeast	________________
Tinea corporis	________________
Hepatitis (contagious)	________________
Bacterial conjunctivitis	________________
HIV	________________
Pyrogenic granuloma	________________
Onychophagy	________________
Onychocriptosis	________________
Corregations	________________

Melanonychia ______________________

Leukoderma ______________________

Scabies ______________________

Pediculosis capitis ______________________

Pseudomonas aerations/mold ______________________

Rosacia ______________________

Eczema ______________________

Steatoma ______________________

Keratoma ______________________

Keratosis ______________________

Tinea pedis ______________________

Chloasma ______________________

Malignant melanoma ______________________

Pityriasis (dandruff) ______________________

Pityriasis steatoides ______________________

Onychorrhexis ______________________

Onychocryptosis ______________________

Onycholysis ______________________

Onychomadesis ______________________

Nail psoriasis ______________________

Paronychia ______________________

Onychomycosis ______________________

Mole ______________________

Tinea unguium ______________________

Psoriasis ______________________

WORD REVIEW

allergens
allergic contact dermatitis
chronic
corrosives
disposable gloves
formaldehyde
irritant contact dermatitis
Malassezia
MSDS
natural latex
neoprene
nickel
nitrile
polyethylene
polyurethane
PVA
Sensitization
Sensitized
Sensitizers
vinyl

Date ______________

Rating ______________

Text Pages 55–72

Chapter 6 The Growth and Structure of Hair

WHY WE NEED HAIR

1. Matching: Match the terms on the left with their correct descriptions on the right.

________ 1. Julius Caesar	A. cutting his hair was considered his downfall
________ 2. 1960s/USA	B. noticed that eunuchs never lost their hair
________ 3. Aristotle	C. had absolutely no hair on their bodies
________ 4. historical Japanese women	D. their hair was considered to be the least important body part
________ 5. Samson	E. wore a laurel wreath to hide his baldness
	F. hair was important for survival
	G. long hair was a political statement
	H. immortal spirit was thought to be located in their hair

STRUCTURES OF THE SCALP

2. How many hair follicles are on the scalp?

____

3. A. In follicle formation, in what direction does the epidermis grow in order to create the canal called the follicle?

____

B. The follicle canal wraps itself tightly around, and almost completely surrounds, a piece of

______________.

C. How many times does follicle formation happen on the average body?

____

4. Label the stages of the origin of follicle and hair.

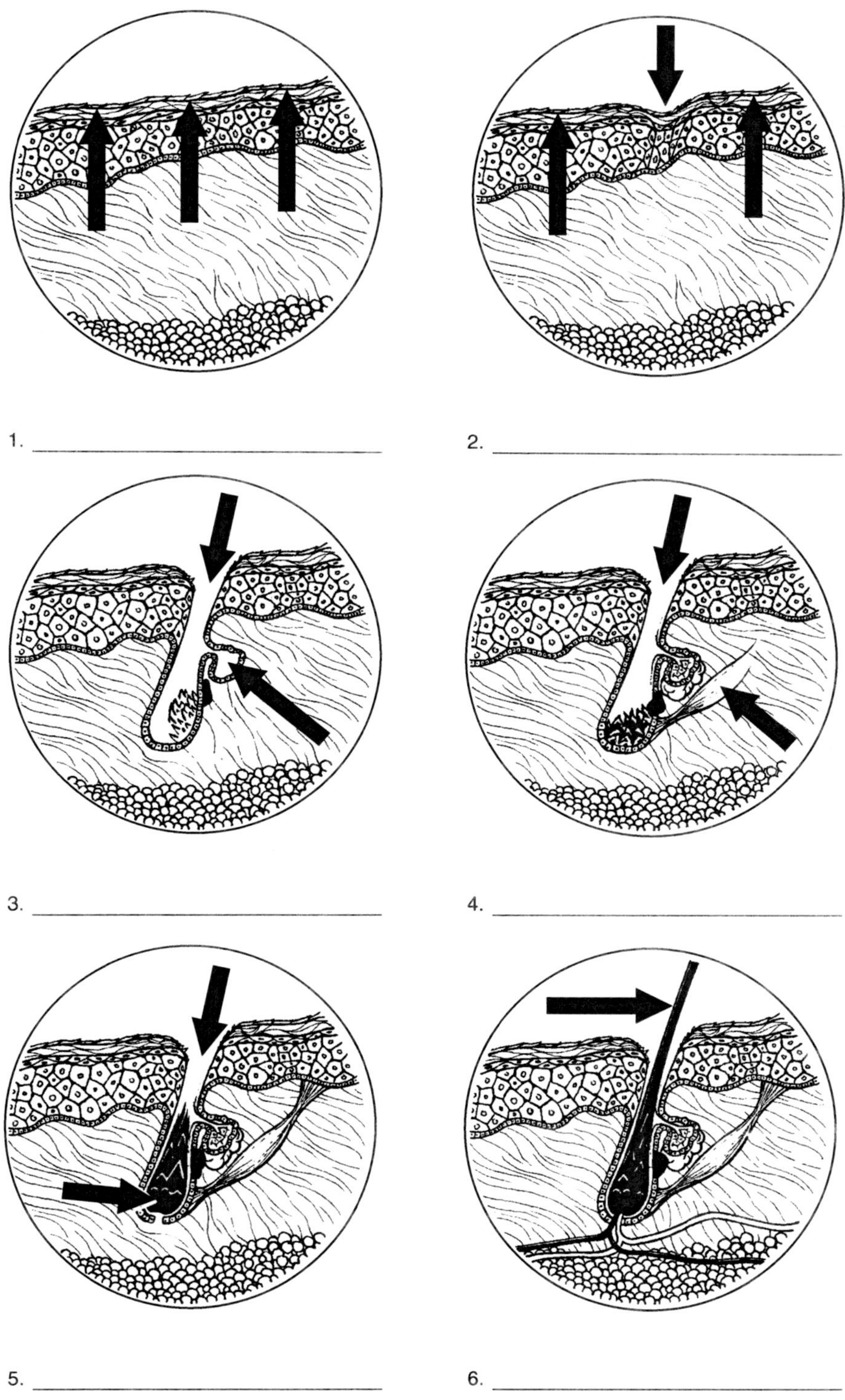

5. Identify the name of the cone-shaped piece of dermis tissue that bulges into the follicle canal.

______

6. A. What supplies oxygen and nutrients to the follicle canal?

____

B. These (the answer to question 6A) remain attached to the hair ________________.

7. A. Special types of cells from which hair grows are called ________________.

B. The cells named in question 7A come from a small bulge that is located directly under the

________________.

C. The cytoplasm of these new cells is completely replaced by a protein called ________________.

This process is known as ________________.

D. Identify where these cells go as more of them are made.

____

8. Identify when the cells in question 7A die.

____

9. The type of cell that contains NO cytoplasm or nucleus is a/an ________________ cell.

10. A. Identify the gland that secretes sebum.

____

B. Sebum is secreted into the ________________.

C. How much sebum is made by the body?

____

D. What does sebum do for the hair and skin?

____

11. A. The name of the bulge attached to the follicle that causes goosebumps is the

________________.

B. List two purposes of the arrector pili muscle.

1. ______________________________

2. ______________________________

12. Identify the parts of the skin and hair shown in the illustration.

Hair shaft or stem–that part of the hair that extends wholly above the skin.

STRUCTURE OF HAIR

13. Identification Match: Using the terms listed below, match the characteristics with the correct layer of hair.

medulla
cortex
cuticle

Characteristics:

______________ 1. made up of angular-shaped keratin cells

______________ 2. this layer is an "empty" air space, not involved in salon services

______________ 3. protects the other two layers

______________ 4. the cells overlap like roof shingles

______________ 5. it's common for very fine and naturally blond hair to lack this layer

________________ 6. the innermost portion of the hair shaft

________________ 7. color pigment is found in this layer

________________ 8. this layer is lacking in very fine hair

________________ 9. makes up 90% of the hair's total weight

________________ 10. pH and hot temperature can loosen it

________________ 11. made up of transparent, scale-like cells

________________ 12. gives hair its strength and elasticity

SUBFIBERS AND PHYSICAL PROPERTIES OF HAIR

14. Wet hair can be stretched up to ________________ % and return to its original length.

15. Matching: Match the terms on the left with their correct descriptions on the right.

________ 1. protein	A. The reduced form of cystine
________ 2. cystine	B. the shape of a straight protein
________ 3. peptide bond	C. made of long chains of amino acids
________ 4. helix	D. the hollow center of a keratin cell
________ 5. amino acids	E. The oxidized form of cysteine
________ 6. disulfide bond	F. also called end bond
________ 7. cysteine	G. 18 different types make proteins of hair
________ 8. polypeptides	H. the shape of a coiled protein
	I. long polypeptide chains
	J. on average, it contains 10,985 amino acids
	K. The side bond between two cysteine sulfur atoms

16. A. List the three different types of side bonds.

    1. ____________________
    2. ____________________
    3. ____________________

    B. List the three salon services to which side bonds are essential.

    1. ____________________
    2. ____________________
    3. ____________________

    C. What type of side bond is easily broken by water or heat?

    ____

    D. What type of side bond is dependant on pH?

    ____

    E. These are the strongest side bonds in hair and are not broken by water or heat.

    ____

    F. How does cysteine form cystine?

    ____

17. Micro fibrils are made of ____________________.

18. Macro fibrils are made of ____________________.

19. Fibrils are made of ____________________.

20. Fibrils are the cells of the hair's ____________________ layer.

21. A. How many amino acids make up the protein structures of hair?

    ____

B. The most abundant amino acid in hair is ______________________, which makes up

______________________ % of hair.

22. What is the F-layer?

____

____

____

WORD REVIEW

amino acids
arrector pili muscle
cortex
cuticle
cysteine
cystine
dermal papilla
dermis
disulfide bonds
end bonds
fibrils
follicle
hair bulb
helix
hydrogen bonds
keratin
keratinization
macro fibrils
medulla
18 methyl eicosanoic acid (18MEA)
micro fibrils
polypeptides
salt bonds
sebaceous/oil gland
sebum
side bonds
stem cells

Date ____________________

Rating ____________________

Text Pages 73–90

Chapter 7 The Properties of Hair

GROWTH CYCLES

1. Identification Match: Using the terms listed below, match the characteristics with the correct hair growth phase.

anagen phase
catagen phase
telogen phase

Characteristics:

____________________ 1. the resting stage

____________________ 2. new keratinized cells are manufactured

____________________ 3. germ cells are made

____________________ 4. cells stop making color pigments

____________________ 5. this cycle lasts approximately three to six months

____________________ 6. this cycle generally lasts three to five years

____________________ 7. the old hair is usually shed

____________________ 8. the growth cycle

____________________ 9. the follicle canal shrinks

HAIR TYPES

2. A. List three places where vellus hair can be found on adults.

1. ____________________

2. ____________________

3. ____________________

B. Identify the missing layer of hair in vellus hair.

____

C. Vellus hair is usually replaced by thicker ______________________ hair.

D. Women retain ______________________% more vellus hair than men.

E. List three characteristics that describe vellus hair.

1. ____

2. ____

3. ____

3. A. List three ways in which terminal hair is different from vellus hair.

1. ____

2. ____

3. ____

B. List two types of primary terminal hair.

1. ____

2. ____

C. List six types of secondary terminal hair.

1. ____

2. ____

3. ____

4. ____

5. ____

6. ____

4. Does one hair follicle make only one type of hair, or can one follicle produce both vellus and terminal hair? Explain.

____

____

NORMAL HAIR LOSS AND GROWTH RATE

5. Fill in the correct percentage of hair in each of the following hair phases.

Phase:	**Percentage:**
Anagen	______________
Catagen	______________
Telogen	______________

6. On average, there are about ______________ hairs on the scalp.

7. How many hairs, on average, are lost each day?

____

8. A. How fast per day does hair grow on:

   1. ____

   2. ____

   B. The answer to question 8A means that ______________ hair grows faster than ______________ hair.

   C. How long does it take for a new hair to emerge after a hair is pulled from the scalp?

   ____

   D. On the following list, place an *F* next to the ONE item that accurately states when hair grows *faster*. Place an *S* next to the ONE item that accurately states when hair grows *more slowly*.

   __________ at night

   __________ after cutting the hair

____________ during pregnancy

____________ in November

____________ in the summer

____________ after shaving

____________ during menstrual cycle

____________ during the day

9. Define *bed-hair*.

____

10. Define *shed-hair*.

____

11. Define *elliptical*.

____

12. The more elliptical a person's hair, the ________________________ the hair. The less elliptical, the ________________________ the hair.

13. A. What percent of its normal dry weight in water can hair absorb?

____

B. What percent of its weight can hair absorb from moisture in the air?

____

C. Added water causes the hair to swell an additional ________________________ % of its diameter.

14. A. Define *hair body*.

____

B. List six body characteristics of hair.

1. ______________________________

2. ______________________________

3. ______________________________

4. ______________________________

5. ______________________________

6. ______________________________

15. A. List two types of melanin.

1. ______________________________

2. ______________________________

B. Identify which type of melanin gives hair yellowish-blond tones.

____

C. Identify which type of melanin gives hair brown to black shades.

____

16. The special cells that make melanin are called ______________.

17. In which layer of the hair is melanin found?

____

18. List three factors that determine all natural hair colors.

1. ______________________________

2. ______________________________

3. ______________________________

19. Explain the difference between the melanin granules of hair that is black in color and the melanin granules of blond hair.

____

20. What does lightening do to melanin granules?

____

21. A. When hair turns gray, it means a decrease in the number of ____________________.

B. This "graying" also means that less melanin is made by the ____________________.

C. List two hair growth phases in which melanin production stops.

1. ____

2. ____

22. A. Define *hair density*.

____

B. What is the average number of hairs per square inch?

____

C. List three factors that cause a DECREASE in hair density.

1. ____

2. ____

3. ____

23. Explain the two different ways in which hair texture can vary.

1. ____

2. ____

24. After each percentage listed below, write in the name of the element that represents that particular percentage of the hair.

Phase:	Percentage:
5%	____________
6%	____________
17%	____________
21%	____________
51%	____________

25. List seven factors that influence hair growth.

1. ____________
2. ____________
3. ____________
4. ____________
5. ____________
6. ____________
7. ____________

HAIR LOSS TREATMENTS

26. A. What are the two drugs that are approved by the FDA to stimulate hair growth?

1. ____________
2. ____________

B. List these same two drugs and the brand names under which they are sold.

1. ____________
2. ____________

C. What is another name for male pattern baldness and what causes it?

____

____

AMINO ACIDS AND NUTRITION

27. Why is it so important that the essential amino acids be included in our diet?

____

28. Why don't the nonessential amino acids need to be in our diet?

____

29. What are complete proteins?

____

30. What are complimentary foods?

____

____

31. List four examples of complimentary foods.

    1. ____

    2. ____

    3. ____

    4. ____

32. What is the only prescription drug approved by the FDA to suppress hair growth?

____

WORD REVIEW

amino acids
anagen phase
bed-hair
carbon
catagen phase
COHNS elements
complete proteins
complimentary foods
diameter
elliptical
essential amino acids
eumelanin
Finasteride/Propecia
germ cells
hair body
hair density
hydrogen
melanin
melanocytes
Minoxidil/Rogaine
nitrogen
nonessential amino acids
oxygen
phaeomelanin
pigment density
primary terminal hairs
secondary terminal hairs
shed-hair
sulfur
telogen
terminal hair
trace elements
vellus hair

Date ______________________

Rating ______________________

Text Pages 91–102

Chapter 8 General Chemistry

1. Why is chemistry called the "central science"?

____

2. List nine examples of salon services that rely on the use of chemicals.

   1. ____
   2. ____
   3. ____
   4. ____
   5. ____
   6. ____
   7. ____
   8. ____
   9. ____

3. What is chemistry?

____

4. List and define the two main branches of chemistry.

   1. ____
   2. ____

5. What does the term organic mean?

____

6. What is matter?

____

____

7. What are elements?

____

____

____

____

8. What are the smallest particles of an element that retain the properties of that element?

____

9. What are the structural units of the elements that make up matter?

____

10. How are the various elements different from each other?

____

MOLECULES

11. A. What are molecules?

____

B. What are the two types of molecules?

1. _______________

2. _______________

C. What is the difference between an elemental molecule and a compound molecule the two types of molecules in question 11B?

____

____

STATES OF MATTER

12. A. List the three states of matter.

1. ____

2. ____

3. ____

B. What are the three states of matter of water?

1. ____

2. ____

3. ____

PHYSICAL AND CHEMICAL PROPERTIES

13. List seven physical properties of matter.

1. ____

2. ____

3. ____

4. ____

5. ____

6. ____

7. ____

14. A. What are the chemical properties of matter?

____

____

B. List two examples of the chemical properties of matter.

1. ____

2. ____

15. A. Define a physical change, and explain how it is different from a chemical change.

____

____

B. Give four examples of a physical change.

1. ____

2. ____

3. ____

4. ____

16. A. Define a chemical change, and explain how it is different from a physical change.

____

____

B. List three examples of a chemical change.

1. ____

2. ____

3. ____

PURE SUBSTANCES, COMPOUNDS, AND MIXTURES

17. A. What are pure substances?

____

B. List the two types of pure substances, and give an example of each.

1. _______________

2. _______________

18. Give an example of a mixture of gases.

____

19. Give an example of a physical mixture of solids.

____

20. What two things distinguish between solutions, suspensions, and emulsions?

1. _______________

2. _______________

SOLUTIONS

21. A. What are solutions?

____

B. What is a solute?

____

C. What is a solvent?

____

D. What are miscible liquids?

____

E. Give an example of a pair of miscible liquids.

____

F. What are immiscible liquids?

____

G. Give an example of a pair of immiscible liquids.

____

22. Indicate to the left if the descriptions below are those of solutions, emulsions, or suspensions.

__________________ A. mayonnaise

__________________ B. contain particles the size of a small molecule that are invisible to the naked eye

__________________ C. salt water

__________________ D. contain particles large enough to be visible to the naked eye

__________________ E. do not separate on standing

__________________ F. are not usually transparent and may be colored

__________________ G. oil and vinegar salad dressing

__________________ H. mixtures of two immiscible liquids held together by an emulsifying agent

__________________ I. are usually transparent, although they may be colored

__________________ J. should be stable for at least three years

WORD REVIEW

atoms
chemical change
chemical compounds
chemistry
compound molecules
elemental molecules
elements
emulsifier
emulsions
inorganic chemistry
matter
mixtures
organic chemistry
physical change
pure substance
solutions
states of matter
suspensions

Date ______________________

Rating ______________________

Text Pages 103–112

Chapter 9 Advanced Chemistry

1. Indicate if the pH values listed below are acidic, neutral, or alkaline.

______________________ A. pH 7

______________________ B. pH 14

______________________ C. pH 3

______________________ D. pH 8

2. A. What is an ion?

____

B. What is an anion?

____

C. What is a cation?

____

3. A. What two ions are produced as a result of the natural ionization of water?

1. ____

2. ____

B. Indicate if the ions in question 3.A are acidic or alkaline.

1. ____

2. ____

C. Why is the pH of pure water neutral?

D. What is the pH of pure alcohol?

THE pH SCALE

4. List four terms that are used to describe pH.

    1.

    2.

    3.

    4.

5. What does the pH scale measure?

6. What is pH?

7. Why do scientists use scientific notation?

8. The number 1×10^{-7} is expressed in scientific notation. What is the same number expressed as a decimal?

9. What does the term *logarithm* mean?

____

10. A pH of 8 is how many times more alkaline than a pH of 7?

____

11. A pH of 9 is how many times more alkaline than a pH of 7?

____

12. Indicate if the descriptions below apply to acids or alkalis.

______________ A. the hydrogen ion

______________ B. sodium hydroxide

______________ C. contract and harden the hair

______________ D. the hydroxide ion

______________ E. taste sour or tart

______________ F. taste bitter

______________ G. (H^+)

______________ H. soften and swell the hair

______________ I. (OH^-)

13. Why are some acids and alkalis stronger than others?

____

____

____

14. What happens when acids and alkalis are mixed together in equal proportions?

____

OXIDATION-REDUCTION (REDOX) REACTIONS

15. What are exothermic reactions?

____

16. Give an example of an exothermic reaction.

____

____

17. Give two examples of slow oxidation reactions.

1. ____

2. ____

18. What is combustion?

____

19. Indicate if the descriptions below apply to oxidation or reduction.

_______________ A. when oxygen is combined with a substance

_______________ B. when oxygen is removed from a substance

_______________ C. hydrogen peroxide

_______________ D. results from the loss of hydrogen

_______________ E. results from the addition of hydrogen

_______________ F. permanent-wave solution

_______________ G. permanent-wave neutralizers

WORD REVIEW

acid/acids/acidic
alkali/alkalis/alkaline
anions
base/basic
cations
decimal
exponent
exponential notation
hydrogen ions (H^+)
hydroxide ions (OH^-)
ions
logarithm
neutral
oxidation
pH
reduction

Date ____________________

Rating ____________________

Text Pages 113–140

Chapter 10 Shampoos, Conditioners, and Styling Aids

1. A. Water is a polar molecule. What does that mean?

____

B. What is the result of hydrogen bonding in water?

____

C. What causes hydrogen bonding in water?

____

____

2. Indicate if the statements below apply to water or oil.

____________________ A. acts as a solvent for most other ionic substances

____________________ B. acts as a solvent for substances that have the ability to hydrogen bond

____________________ C. is lipophilic

____________________ D. is hydrophilic

____________________ E. is nonpolar

____________________ F. is lipophobic

____________________ G. is polar

3. How do surfactants form an emulsion?

____

____

4. A. What is the Latin meaning of *detergent?*

____

B. What is the most traditional type of detergent?

____

5. A. Identify the two ingredients used to make soaps.

1. ____

2. ____

B. List four oils used in making soap.

1. ____

2. ____

3. ____

4. ____

C. Discuss two negative effects soap has on the hair and skin.

1. ____

2. ____

6. A. The term surfactant is a contraction for ____________________.

B. Surfactants work between the surfaces of two substances. Name them.

1. ____

2. ____

C. The boundary where oil meets water is called the ____________________.

7. A. Explain how shampoo foaming/lathering occurs.

____

B. Is a large quantity of foam a sign of a good quality shampoo? Check one:

__________ yes

__________ no

C. Explain the reaction between foam and sebum/oils.

____

8. Identify seven considerations when choosing the type of surfactant to use.

1. ____

2. ____

3. ____

4. ____

5. ____

6. ____

7. ____

9. Matching: Match the terms on the left with their correct descriptions on the right.

__________	1. cationic	A.	surfactants that have neither a positive nor a negative charge
__________	2. saponins	B.	antibacterial surfactants with a positive charge
__________	3. nonionic	C.	surfactants that are both positively and negatively charged
__________	4. anionic	D.	the most widely used surfactants with a negative charge
__________	5. amphoteric	E.	the only surfactant found in nature

EMULSIONS

10. List eight of the different functions and purposes that surfactants serve.

    1. ______________________________

    2. ______________________________

    3. ______________________________

    4. ______________________________

    5. ______________________________

    6. ______________________________

    7. ______________________________

    8. ______________________________

11. A. What is an emulsion?

    ____

    ____

    B. What are the two most common types of emulsions?

    1. ______________________________

    2. ______________________________

    C. Indicate if the statements below apply to oil-in-water (O/W) or water-in-oil (W/O) emulsions.

    ____________ 1. Droplets of oil are dispersed in water.

    ____________ 2. Micelles surround droplets of water.

    ____________ 3. Surfactant "heads" point in and their "tails" point out.

    ____________ 4. Micelles surround droplets of oil.

________________________ 5. Surfactant “tails” point in and their “heads” point out.

________________________ 6. Water is the continuous or external phase.

________________________ 7. Oil is the continuous or external phase.

________________________ 8. Water is the discontinuous or internal phase.

________________________ 9. Oil is the discontinuous or internal phase.

________________________ 10. he most common emulsions used in a salon.

________________________ 11. Droplets of water are dispersed in oil.

D. What are multiple-phase emulsions?

____

____

12. Fill-in: Using the following list of words, fill in the correct word for each statement.

Word List:

anionic	opacifier
chelator	pearling agent
coloring/fragrance	preservative
conditioner	saponins
detangler	surfactant
emulsion	thickener
foam builders	water

Statements:

________________________ 1. cationic surfactant that coats the hair to improve wet combing

________________________ 2. covers up cloudiness or unattractive colors

________________________ 3. the solvent that makes up 45%–75% of a shampoo’s content

________________________ 4. makes up less than 1% of shampoo ingredients, but sells 90% of all shampoos

________________________ 5. adds shine and moisture to the hair

________________________ 6. gives shampoo a pearlescent texture

____________________ 7. three or four of these are in shampoo to make up 30%–40% of its content

____________________ 8. prevents film from depositing on the hair shaft

____________________ 9. their purpose is to create large amounts of thick, creamy-feeling bubbles

____________________ 10. plant gums and synthetic polymers are two types

____________________ 11. inhibits bacteria growth

CONDITIONER CHEMISTRY

13. List 12 possible causes of hair damage.

1. ____
2. ____
3. ____
4. ____
5. ____
6. ____
7. ____
8. ____
9. ____
10. ____
11. ____
12. ____

14. List four characteristics of damaged hair.

1. ____
2. ____

3. ____________________

4. ____________________

15. Identify nine ways hair conditioners can improve hair.

1. ____________________

2. ____________________

3. ____________________

4. ____________________

5. ____________________

6. ____________________

7. ____________________

8. ____________________

9. ____________________

16. Identification Match: Using the terms listed below, match the characteristics with the correct conditioning chemicals.

Key
protein and protein derivatives
humectants
moisturizers

Characteristics:

____________ 1. lanolin, mineral oil, and cholesterol are examples

____________ 2. hydrolized ones improve hair strength and elasticity

____________ 3. lanolin, oleic, and stearic acids are examples

____________ 4. oily substances that coat the hair or skin

____________ 5. like sponges, they attract moisture to the skin and scalp

_____________ 6. examples are sodium PCA, sodium lactate, and glycerin

_____________ 7. are long chains containing hundreds of amino acids

17. A. What are fatty alcohols?

____

____

B. List four examples of fatty alcohols.

1. _____________
2. _____________
3. _____________
4. _____________

18. What are silicones?

____

____

19. Why are silicones superior to plain oil?

____

____

STYLING AIDS

20. A. What are the two main types of styling aids?

1. _____________
2. _____________

B. What is the most important ingredient in any setting lotion?

____

21. A. What do the letters SD, in SD alcohol, stand for?

____

B. List the two chemical names for the alcohol that is found in alcoholic beverages.

1. ______________________________

2. ______________________________

C. Why is the alcohol in cosmetic products denatured?

____

____

22. A. What is the major difference between the way setting lotions and hairsprays are used?

____

____

B. What is the major difference between the way setting lotions and hairsprays are formulated?

____

____

23. A. What are volatile organic compounds (VOCs)?

____

B. What are chlorofluorocarbons (CFCs)?

____

____

C. Are CFCs still used in hairspray in the United States? Why or why not?

____

____

24. List 4 reasons why chelating agents, also called sequestrants, are added to shampoos.

1. ______________________________

2. ______________________________

3. ______________________________

4. ______________________________

5. ______________________________

25. What is the name of the fungus that causes dandruff?

____

26. List three anti-fungal agents that are used to treat dandruff.

1. ______________________________

2. ______________________________

3. ______________________________

27. List four types of surfactants that are commonly used in sulfate free shampoos.

1. ______________________________

2. ______________________________

3. ______________________________

4. ______________________________

28. How can 2-in-1 conditioning shampoos clean hair when they contain a conditioner?

____

____

WORD REVIEW

amphoteric
anionic
cationic
chelators
chlorofluorocarbons (CFCs)
coloring conditioner
detanglers
detergent
emulsion
ethyl alcohol
fatty acids
fatty alcohols
foam builders/stabilizers
folklore ingredients
fragrance
humectants
hydrogen bonding
hydrophilic
hydrophobic
interface
inverse micelle
ion
ionic bonds
lipophilic
lipophobic
micelle
moisturizers
negative ions
nonionic
non-polar
molecules
opacifiers
organic acids
pearling agents
photoxidative
effects
positive ions
preservatives
protein
salt bonds
saponins
SD alcohol
seborrhea
silicones
soap
surface tension
surfactants
thickeners
vitamins
volatile alcohols
volatile organic compounds
(VOCs)
wetting

Date ______________________

Rating ______________________

Text Pages 141–166

Chapter 11 Color and Hair Lightening

1. A. People have colored their hair for ______________________ of years.

   B. In what year was the first synthetic dye used?

   ____

THE SOURCE OF COLOR

2. A. The only difference between visible light and all other types of electromagnetic radiation is their

   ______________________.

   B. What is a wavelength?

   ____

   C. Indicate if the statements below apply to long or short wavelengths.

   ______________________ 1. radio waves

   ______________________ 2. have higher frequencies

   ______________________ 3. penetrate deeper

   ______________________ 4. are not as energetic

   ______________________ 5. are more energetic

   ______________________ 6. ultra-violet rays

   ______________________ 7. have lower frequencies

   ______________________ 8. do not penetrate as deeply

   ______________________ 9. infrared rays

   ______________________ 10. X-rays

3. List the six colors the eyes can see.

   1. ______________________________

   2. ______________________________

   3. ______________________________

   4. ______________________________

   5. ______________________________

   6. ______________________________

4. When a person sees a red apple, it means that the red light is being ________________, and all other colors are being ________________.

5. A. Matching: Match the terms on the left with their correct descriptions on the right.

________	1. level of color	A. mixing equal parts of a primary and tertiary color
________	2. secondary colors	B. red, blue, and yellow
________	3. quarternary colors	C. balance of colors
________	4. complementary colors	D. red, green, and brown
________	5. primary colors	E. mixing equal parts of a primary color with an adjacent secondary color
________	6. tone	F. green, violet, and orange
________	7. tertiary colors	G. indicates a color's lightness or darkness
		H. all colors besides primary, secondary, and tertiary colors
		I. white, blue, and red-orange
		J. two colors opposite each other on the color wheel

B. List the three different terms that are used to define the level of color.

   1. ______________________________

2. ______________________________

3. ______________________________

C. What question does the level of color answer?

____

D. Which color is the result of mixing equal parts of all three primary colors with the highest concentration of pigment?

____

E. Which color is the result of mixing equal parts of all three primary colors with the least concentration of pigment?

____

F. List the term that is used to define the tone or hue of color.

____

G. What question does the tone or hue of color answer?

____

H. What colors result from unequal proportions of all three primary colors?

____

I. A natural brown or blond hair color is composed of:

____

J. What is the difference between a natural brown or blond color?

____

6. A. What is melanin?

____

B. What is white hair?

____

C. List two types of melanin.

1. ____

2. ____

D. Of the two in question 6C, the type of melanin that gives hair yellow and red tones is

_______________________.

The type of melanin that gives hair shades from brown to black is _______________________.

7. List three factors that determine natural hair color.

1. ____

2. ____

3. ____

LIGHTENING THE HAIR

8. Explain decolorization.

____

9. Identify two purposes of lighteners.

1. ____

2. ____

10. Decolorizing hair makes it reflect light instead of _______________________ it.

11. Decolorizing hair doesn't just make it lighter. It also makes it _______________________.

12. Darker hair may not lighten beyond what stage?

____

13. What color toner should be used to neutralize orange hair?

____

14. What color toner should be used to neutralize yellow hair?

____

15. List the 10 degrees, or stages, of decolorization from darkest to lightest.

1. ______________________________
2. ______________________________
3. ______________________________
4. ______________________________
5. ______________________________
6. ______________________________
7. ______________________________
8. ______________________________
9. ______________________________
10. ______________________________

16. A. What is the chemical symbol for hydrogen peroxide?

____

B. What is the chemical symbol for water?

____

C. The solution of hydrogen peroxide used in salons is a mixture of what two chemicals?

1. ______________________________
2. ______________________________

D. What do the different volumes of hydrogen peroxide indicate?

____

E. Decomposition of one ounce of 20-volume peroxide yields how many ounces of oxygen gas?

____

F. Decomposition of one ounce of 10-volume peroxide yields how many ounces of oxygen gas?

____

G. List three of the materials that are used to thicken liquid peroxide and make cream developers.

1. ____

2. ____

3. ____

17. Fill in the missing information on the following chart, which compares percentages and volumes of peroxide.

Percentage of hydrogen peroxide in water:	**Peroxide volume/s:**
3	________
________	20
________	30
12	________
________	100

18. A. To prevent premature breakdown, solutions of hydrogen peroxide are acid ________________.

pH AND HAIR LIGHTENING

19. A. What is the pH of most hair lighteners?

____

B. List the two reasons why effective hair lighteners must have an alkaline pH.

1. ______________________________

2. ______________________________

20. A. What is the chemical formula for ammonia?

____

B. From what chemical does ammonia derive its chemical reactivity?

____

C. Why does ammonia have such a strong odor?

____

21. A. What are alkanolamines?

____

B. List two examples of common organic alkalis that are used instead of ammonia.

1. ______________________________

2. ______________________________

C. Indicate if the statements below apply to ammonia or alkanolamines.

______________ 1. an inorganic alkali

______________ 2. large, organic molecules that contain carbon

______________ 3. there is little or no odor

______________ 4. more effective for hair lightening than other alkalizing agents

______________ 5. gaining in popularity because of their low odor

______________ 6. strong, offensive odor

______________ 7. not as effective at lightening the hair

22. Besides melanin, identify two other structures/parts of the hair that are affected by oxidation.

    1. ______________________________

    2. ______________________________

23. A single lightening application can lower the hair's strength by ______________ %.

24. List six symptoms that require a client to see a dermatologist before receiving a chemical service.

    1. ______________________________

    2. ______________________________

    3. ______________________________

    4. ______________________________

    5. ______________________________

    6. ______________________________

25. Define porosity gradients.

    ____

26. Chemical treatments process faster on hair that is located near the ______________. This is because the head gives off ______________. For every 18°F/10°C rise in temperature, the rate of a chemical reaction is ______________.

27. Identify three variables strand testing can help control.

    1. ______________________________

    2. ______________________________

    3. ______________________________

28. Name two hair problems caused by overlapping.

    1. ______________________________

    2. ______________________________

29. Explain what happens if lightener residue is left on the hair.

____

30. List six forms of hair lighteners.

    1. ____
    2. ____
    3. ____
    4. ____
    5. ____
    6. ____

PERSONAL SAFETY

31. To avoid injury when mixing chemicals, you should always follow ________________________ directions/ instructions.

32. List two parts of the body that oxidizers can easily damage.

    1. ____
    2. ____

33. Hair lightening and haircoloring services causes the hair to feel dry and rough and become more hydrophilic and absorb water more easily because it removes what layer of the hair?

____

34. Excessive hair lightening converts cystine into

____

WORD REVIEW

alkanolamines
aminomethylpropanol
ammonia (NH_3)
balance of color
complementary colors
concentration
cream lighteners
decolorizing
density
electromagnetic spectrum
eumelanin
high frequency
hydrogen peroxide (H_2O_2)
inorganic alkali
keratin
laws of color
level of color
lightener
long wavelength
low frequency
melanin
monoethanolamine
organic alkali
overlapping
oxidation
oxidizer
paste lighteners
phaeomelanin
porosity gradients
primary colors
quaternary colors
saturation
secondary colors
short wavelength
tertiary colors
tone or hue of color
visible light
visible spectrum
volume of peroxide
water (H_2O)
white light

Date ______________________

Rating ______________________

Text Pages 167–186

Chapter 12 Haircoloring

1. What are the two main categories of professional haircoloring products marketed for salon use?

   1. ______________________

   2. ______________________

2. A. List the two different types of nonoxidation colors.

   1. ______________________

   2. ______________________

   B. List the two different types of oxidation colors.

   1. ______________________

   2. ______________________

3. List six forms of temporary haircolor.

   1. ______________________

   2. ______________________

   3. ______________________

   4. ______________________

   5. ______________________

   6. ______________________

4. Define *affinity*.

____

5. What does an alkaline pH level do to the hair's cuticle layer?

____

6. Indicate if the statements below apply to nonoxidation colors or oxidation colors.

_______________ 1. contain only one component

_______________ 2. the color in the bottle is the color deposited on the hair

_______________ 3. contain two components

_______________ 4. there is no chemical reaction involved

_______________ 5. are not used directly as they come out of the bottle

_______________ 6. used directly as they come out of the bottle

_______________ 7. deposit stable, direct dyes that have been formed prior to application.

_______________ 8. create a chemical change in the hair

_______________ 9. must be mixed with developer or activator immediately before use

_______________ 10. are not mixed with developer or activator

_______________ 11. the final color is developed, on the hair, during processing

_______________ 12. the change in the hair is only physical

_______________ 13. the color in the original bottle is not the color deposited on the hair

7. Using the following list of words, fill in the correct word for each statement.

Word List:

affinity	primary intermediates
heat	dye solvent
ammonia	toner
metallic dye	enzyme
antioxidant	activator
modifier	viscosity
developer	filler

Statements:

_______________ 1. slows down the oxidizer to allow more time for application

_______________ 2. colors prelightened hair to a delicate shade

_______________ 3. chemically combines with primary intermediates to create complex color blends

_______________ 4. breaks down dye molecules to remove them from the hair

_______________ 5. penetrates broken cuticle and fills small holes in the hair

_______________ 6. the major color-producing chemicals in permanent haircoloring

_______________ 7. accelerates most chemical reactions

_______________ 8. another name for oxidizer

8. A. Indicate if the statements below apply to demi-permanent or permanent color.

_______________ 1. can lighten and deposit color at the same time, and in one process

_______________ 2. will not lighten the natural hair color

_______________ 3. is usually mixed with a lower volume developer

_______________ 4. is usually more alkaline

_______________ 5. is called no lift-deposit, only color

_______________ 6. is usually less alkaline

_______________ 7. is usually mixed with a higher volume developer

B. Identify two actions that permanent oxidation products have on hair.

1. ____

2. ____

C. What are the two reasons that hydrogen peroxide is added to permanent haircolor?

1. ______________________________

2. ______________________________

9. A. What are the two factors that determine the amount of lift in a permanent color?

1. ______________________________

2. ______________________________

B. By what percentage is the final concentration of peroxide in the finished color mixture increased by using double peroxide instead of equal parts?

____

10. Explain how toners differ from permanent haircolor.

____

11. A. Will a haircolor service processed with a machine at 90°F process faster than it would at a normal room temperature of 72°F? If so, how much faster will it process?

____

B. What should a hairstylist do to avoid evaporation when using dry heat?

____

12. A. What are enzymes?

____

____

B. Are enzymes any more effective or less damaging than peroxide? Why or why not?

____

____

13. A. Two types of color removers are dye solvents and ________________________.

    B. Identify three dye solvent ingredients.

    1. ______________________________
    2. ______________________________
    3. ______________________________

    C. List three safety precautions that should be taken when using dye solvents.

    1. ______________________________
    2. ______________________________
    3. ______________________________

NONOXIDATION PERMANENT COLORS

14. Identification Match: Identify the characteristics below as either henna or metallic dye.

Characteristics:

________________________ 1. lead, silver, copper, and nickel

________________________ 2. mixed with water to form a paste

________________________ 3. lawsone makes up 1% of the leaf

________________________ 4. destroys disulfide side bonds in the cortex

________________________ 5. a small, attractive bush

________________________ 6. used in retail, "home use" products

________________________ 7. a vegetable dye

________________________ 8. are not used professionally

________________________ 9. contains tannic acid

__________________ 10. skin can absorb and may cause illness

__________________ 11. if mixed with hydrogen peroxide, can cause hair to melt

__________________ 12. builds up on the hair's surface

HAIRCOLORING SAFETY

15. Open sores or other problems can be determined when you __________________ the scalp and hair.

16. When a hair's porosity differs along its length, it is referred to as a porosity __________________.

17. To avoid problems caused by damaged hair, questions of timing, and/or improper mixing, it is suggested that you perform a/an __________________ test.

18. Scalp heat causes the hair near the scalp to lighten __________________ than the hair near the ends.

19. A. To determine if a client is allergic to a product, a patch or __________________ test should be given.

    B. Identify four allergic reaction symptoms.

    1. __________________
    2. __________________
    3. __________________
    4. __________________

    C. List five places on the body where the symptoms in 19B usually occur.

    1. __________________
    2. __________________
    3. __________________
    4. __________________
    5. __________________

D. Allergic reactions usually begin within ________________hours after exposure.

E. Identify what/who requires cosmetologists to perform patch tests.

____

20. Define *carcinogen*.

____

21. Define *mutagen*.

____

22. Define *teratogen*.

____

23. Allergic reactions to a tinting ingredient occur after a person becomes ________________________ to it.

24. List two types of contact dermatitis.

 1. ____

 2. ____

25. The advanced form of allergic dermatitis is called ________________________.

WORD REVIEW

affinity
allergic contact dermatitis
ammonia
aniline dyes
antioxidant
carcinogen
catalyze
certified dyes
chronic
couplers
developer
direct dyes
dye solvent
eczema
eumelanin
filler
henna
intermediate bases
irritant contact dermatitis
lawsome
demi-permanent colors
melanin
metallic dyes
modifiers
mutagen
nonoxidation colors
oxidation
oxidation colors
oxidizer
patch test
permanent colors
phaeomelanin
predisposition test
primary intermediates
sensitization
sensitizers
strand test
tannic acid
teratogen
toner
viscosity

Date ______________________

Rating ______________________

Text Pages 187–214

Chapter 13 Permanent Waving

HAIR STRUCTURE

1. A. The hair's cortex layer is made up of long chains of amino acid, which are called ______________________.

   B. Identify the four main functions that the cortex provides for the hair.

   1. ______________________
   2. ______________________
   3. ______________________
   4. ______________________

2. Fibrils are made of intertwined ______________, which are made up of bundles of smaller ______________________.

3. Identify two ways polypeptide chains are bound together.

   1. ______________________
   2. ______________________

CHEMICAL BONDS

4. A. List the three types of side bonds that cross-link polypeptide chains together.

   1. ______________________
   2. ______________________
   3. ______________________

   B. What four salon services are made possible only by altering the three side bonds?

   1. ______________________
   2. ______________________

3. ______________________________

4. ______________________________

5. Identification Match: Match the characteristics below with the correct type of bond.

peptide bonds
disulfide bonds
salt bonds
hydrogen bonds

Characteristics:

______________ 1. are sometimes called sulfur bonds

______________ 2. the smallest individual strands in keratin

______________ 3. hair absorbs water and the shaft swells

______________ 4. may contain over 8,000 amino acids

______________ 5. formed by cysteine, a unique amino acid, which makes up 18% of hair

______________ 6. formed between two cystine (**SIS**-teen) amino acids

______________ 7. easily broken by alkaline solutions

______________ 8. also called end bonds

______________ 9. a special type of ionic bond

______________ 10. link long chains of amino acids end to end to make polypeptides

______________ 11. hydrogen from one amino acid is attracted to oxygen from another amino acid

______________ 12. are not broken by heat or water

______________ 13. occurs between the negative and positive charges of amino acids

______________ 14. easily broken simply by wetting the hair with water

6. What are the two changes that take place in the permanent waving process?

   1. ______________________________

   2. ______________________________

7. In permanent waving, what determines the size and type of curl?

____

8. Indicate if the statements below apply to a croquignole or a spiral perm wrap.

______________ 1. Hair is wrapped from the ends to the scalp in overlapping, concentric layers.

______________ 2. Hair is wrapped at an angle other than perpendicular to the length of the rod.

______________ 3. Each layer of hair partially overlaps the preceding layer.

______________ 4. Produces a tighter curl at the ends and a larger curl at the scalp.

______________ 5. This wrapping method produces a uniform curl from the scalp to the ends.

______________ 6. Overlapping is uniform along the length of the rod.

______________ 7. The effective size of the rod increases with each overlapping layer.

______________ 8. The effective size of the rod remains constant along the entire strand of hair.

______________ 9. Hair is wrapped at an angle perpendicular to the length of the rod.

______________ 10. Each layer of hair is wrapped on top of the previous layer.

______________ 11. Longer, thicker hair benefits most from this effect.

THE CHEMISTRY OF PERMANENT WAVING

9. What effect do highly alkaline solutions have on the hair?

____

10. Explain the action of a reducing agent.

___

11. A. How does permanent-waving solution break disulfide bonds?

___

___

B. What determines the strength of the permanent-waving solution?

___

C. What should the strength of the perm solution correspond to?

___

D. What should the alkalinity of the perm solution correspond to?

___

___

12. Indicate if the statements below apply to alkaline waves, true acid waves, acid balanced waves, or all acid waves.

___ A. The activator tube contains glyceryl monothioglycolate.

___ B. Ammonium thioglycolate is the primary reducing agent.

___ C. They process at room temperature.

___ D. They were first introduced in the early 70s.

___ E. They were first developed in 1941.

___ F. They have a pH between 7.8 and 8.2.

___ G. They are also known as cold waves.

___ H. They require the added heat of a hair dryer to accelerate processing.

___ I. They aren't really acidic.

______________________ J. Most of these waves are endothermic.

______________________ K. Glyceryl monothioglycolate is the primary reducing agent.

______________________ L. They have a pH between 9.0 and 9.6.

______________________ M. They have a pH between 4.5 and 7.0.

______________________ N. Repeated exposure is known to cause allergic sensitivity in some individuals.

13. How can a true acid wave, with a pH under 7.0, cause the hair to swell?

____

____

14. A. Define *porosity*.

____

B. What layer of the hair determines porosity?

____

C. Types of hair that are not very porous are normal and ______________________.

D. List three causes of cuticle damage.

1. ____

2. ____

3. ____

E. The greater the cuticle damage, the ______________________ the porosity.

F. Porosity is best evaluated on clean, ______________________ hair by sliding a hair between your fingers from its ______________________ toward the ______________________.

G. Normal/resistant hair feels ______________________ while damaged hair feels ______________________.

15. List two oxidizers found in powdered neutralizers.

1. ______________________________

2. ______________________________

16. Damage from permanents may not appear until several hours later and includes chemical

______________________ .

17. Indicate if the statements below apply to exothermic waves, endothermic waves, or no ammonia waves.

______________________ 1. The activator tube contains an oxidizing agent.

______________________ 2. They require heat from a hair dryer to process properly.

______________________ 3. They will not process properly at room temperature.

______________________ 4. They contain alkanolamines.

______________________ 5. They release heat to the surroundings.

______________________ 6. They absorb heat from the surroundings.

______________________ 7. The solution becomes hot after adding the activator.

______________________ 8. They are gaining in popularity because of their low odor.

PERMANENT-WAVE PROCESSING

18. A. What determines the amount of processing in permanent waving?

____

B. Does processing a permanent wave twice as long process it twice as much?

____

C. When does most of the processing take place?

____

D. Will processing the hair more always result in more curl?

E. When is a thorough saturation of the hair especially important?

NEUTRALIZATION

19. A. List the two functions of proper neutralization.

1.

2.

B. What is the chemical reaction involved in permanent wave neutralization?

C. List three types of permanent-wave neutralizers.

1.

2.

3.

D. How does neutralization rebuild the disulfide bonds that are broken by permanent waving solution?

E. Is a liquid neutralizer absolutely necessary in permanent waving?

WAVE SAFETY

20. A. List two perm ingredients that cause unpleasant odors.

    1. ______________________________

    2. ______________________________

    B. Explain why perms often smell like rotten eggs.

    ____

    C. To mask the odor of perms, manufacturers often add ____________.

    D. Is a nice-smelling product safer than one with an unpleasant odor?

    ____

    ____

    ____

21. List six permanent wave safety precautions.

    1. ______________________________

    2. ______________________________

    3. ______________________________

    4. ______________________________

    5. ______________________________

    6. ______________________________

22. List 11 possible reasons for perm failures.

    1. ______________________________

    2. ______________________________

3. ______________________________

4. ______________________________

5. ______________________________

6. ______________________________

7. ______________________________

8. ______________________________

9. ______________________________

10. ______________________________

11. ______________________________

WORD REVIEW

acid balanced waves
alkaline waves/cold waves
alkanolamines
aminomethylpropanol (AMP)
ammonia
ammonium thioglycolate (ATG)
cortex
croquignole perms
disulfide bonds
endothermic waves
exothermic waves
fibrils
fixative
hydrogen bonds
hydrogen peroxide
ionic bonds
ions keratin
macro fibrils
micro fibrils
monoethanolamine (MEA)
neutralizer
no ammonia waves
organic alkali
oxidizer
peptide bonds
polypeptide
porosity
reducing agents
reduction
salt bonds
shape
spiral perms
thioglycolic acid/thio
true acid waves

Date ______________________

Rating ______________________

Text Pages 215–230

Chapter 14 Chemical Hair Relaxers and Soft Curl Permanents

HAIR RELAXING CHEMISTRY

1. Hair contains millions of ______________________ chains.

2. List three types of side bonds.

   1. ______________________

   2. ______________________

   3. ______________________

3. Matching: Match the terms on the left with their correct descriptions on the right.

________ 1. coarse hair	A. red and black hair usually has a higher content of this
________ 2. sulfur	B. absorbs solutions faster than normal hair
________ 3. dense hair	C. has a larger diameter than normal/average hair
________ 4. fine hair	D. also called metallic dye
________ 5. resistant hair	E. numerous follicles clustered closely together
________ 6. porous hair	F. very few hair follicles on the scalp
	G. has a smaller diameter than normal/average hair
	H. hair's ability to stretch without breaking
	I. cuticle scales are very close together

EXCESSIVELY CURLY HAIR

4. A. What race of people have extremely curly hair?

____

B. What type of hair do African-Americans have?

____

C. List three unique properties of extremely curly hair.

1. ______________________________

2. ______________________________

3. ______________________________

D. Where does extremely curly hair usually break? Why?

____

____

5. What is meant by "reduced hair"?

____

6. List two forms of physical action.

1. ______________________________

2. ______________________________

7. Reduced hair lacks strength and is very ______________.

8. A. The goal of permanent waving is to make naturally ______________ hair ______________.

B. The goal of chemical relaxing is to make naturally ______________ hair ______________.

9. A. Define *viscosity*.

____

B. Explain why relaxers have a higher viscosity than permanent-wave solutions.

____

10. Explain what can happen if the chemical relaxer is left on the hair too long.

____

11. What are the two most common types of chemical hair relaxers?

1. _______________

2. _______________

THIO RELAXERS

12. A. List three unique differences between thio relaxers and thio permanent waves.

1. _______________

2. _______________

3. _______________

B. How do the chemical reactions of thio relaxers compare with those in permanent waving?

____

____

13. A. What is the chemical reaction involved in neutralizers used with thio relaxers?

____

B. How do thio relaxer neutralizers compare to permanent-waving neutralizers?

____

____

14. A. What is a soft curl permanent?

____

____

B. How do the chemicals used in soft curl permanents compare to thio permanent waves?

____

HYDROXIDE RELAXERS

15. A. List four different types of hydroxide relaxers.

    1. ____

    2. ____

    3. ____

    4. ____

B. What is the active ingredient in all hydroxide relaxers?

____

C. How many times more alkaline than the hair is a hydroxide relaxer with a pH of 13.0?

____

____

____

____

E. How is the chemical reaction of hydroxide relaxers different from that of thio relaxers?

____

F. How do hydroxide relaxers work? What is the process called?

____

____

____

HYDROXIDE NEUTRALIZATION

16. A. How is the neutralization of hydroxide relaxers different from that of permanent-waving neutralizers?

B. When neutralizing a hydroxide relaxer, what is neutralized?

C. How are lanthionine bonds different from disulfide bonds?

METAL HYDROXIDE RELAXERS

17. A. List the three different types of metal hydroxide relaxers.

1.
2.
3.

B. List two types of relaxers that are sometimes sold as "no-mix, no lye" relaxers.

1.
2.

C. What type of relaxer is usually sold as "no lye"?

D. What is the active ingredient in all hydroxide relaxers?

E. Are "no lye" relaxers compatible with thio permanents and thio relaxers? Why or why not?

____

____

BASE AND NO-BASE FORMULAS

18. A. What is base cream?

____

____

B. What is a no-base relaxer?

____

____

19. A. Thio relaxers should never be used on hair previously straightened with a/an

_______________ relaxer.

B. List two other names for sodium hydroxide.

1. ____

2. ____

C. Identify the pH level of sodium hydroxide relaxers.

____

D. A sodium hydroxide relaxer should never be used on hair previously straightened with a/an

_______________.

20. A. Identify an example of a low pH reducing agent.

____

B. The pH of a low pH reducing agent is between _______________ and

_______________.

C. List two types of hair recommended for low pH relaxers.

1. ______________________________

2. ______________________________

D. Low pH relaxers are less effective on hair that is ______________________.

E. Compared to regular relaxers, a low pH relaxer's effect on the scalp and hair is ______________________

HAIR RELAXING SAFETY

19. List seven chemical relaxing safety precautions.

1. ______________________________

2. ______________________________

3. ______________________________

4. ______________________________

5. ______________________________

6. ______________________________

7. ______________________________

WORD REVIEW

ammonia
ammonium thioglycolate
base cream
caustic soda
coarse/strong hair
dense hair
disulfide bonds
elasticity test
fine hair
guanidine carbonate
guanidine hydroxide relaxers
hydrogen bonds
hydrogen peroxide
hydroxide neutralizers
hydroxide relaxers (OH^-)
ionic bonds
lanthionine bonds
lanthionization
lithium hydroxide lye
metal hydroxide relaxers
neutralizer
no-base
no-lye
peptide bonds
porosity test
porous hair
potassium hydroxide
reduced state
reduction reactions
resistant hair
shape
side bonds
sodium bisulfite
sodium hydroxide
soft curl permanents
strand test
thio neutralizers
thio relaxers
thioglycolic acid
viscosity

Date ______________________

Rating ______________________

Text Pages 231–242

Chapter 15 Salon Health and Safety

THE IMPORTANCE OF WORKING SAFELY

1. What is a chemical?

____

2. Why are people afraid of chemicals?

____

THE RULES OF WORKING SAFELY

3. Explain the "overexposure principle."

____

____

____

4. Identify who is responsible for proper use and safe handling of chemicals in a salon.

____

5. List three ways to reduce chemical exposure to safe levels.

   1. ____

   2. ____

   3. ____

6. A. The letters OSHA stand for (Occupational Safety and Health Administration).

B. Identify the type of government OSHA represents.

Check one:

_______ local government

_______ state government

_______ federal government

C. List the names of two OSHA regulations.

1. ______________________________

2. ______________________________

D. Describe three purposes of the above regulations.

1. ______________________________

2. ______________________________

3. ______________________________

7. A. The letters MSDS stand for:

____

B. List seven items MSDSs can tell you.

1. ______________________________

2. ______________________________

3. ______________________________

4. ______________________________

5. ______________________________

6. ______________________________

7. ______________________________

C. Identify where an MSDS can be obtained.

____

8. A. Identify four problems caused by improperly stored chemicals.

1. ____

2. ____

3. ____

4. ____

B. List three elements that adversely affect products.

1. ____

2. ____

3. ____

C. Flammable products must be stored away from sources of flame and ____________________.

D. Hydrogen peroxide can explode violently if it is stored in ____________________.

9. A. Identify three ways chemicals can enter your body.

1. ____

2. ____

3. ____

B. These three means of entry are called "routes of ____________________."

10. A. Overexposure for short periods of time results in "short-term" or ____________________ effects.

B. How long is "short-term" considered to be?

____

11. A. Overexposure for long periods of time results in "long-term" or ____________________effects.

B. Long-term effects begin after several ______________________ of repeated overexposure.

12. A. What happens when chlorine bleach is mixed with ammonia or an acid?

____

____

B. What happens when the activator tube from an acid-balanced permanent is mixed with the neutralizer instead of the waving lotion?

____

____

C. What happens when oxidizers are mixed with alkaline chemicals or stored in metal containers?

____

____

13. List nine early warning signs of chemical overexposure.

1. ____

2. ____

3. ____

4. ____

5. ____

6. ____

7. ____

8. ____

9. ____

14. Identify two sources that tell you how to safely handle chemicals.

    1. ______________________________

    2. ______________________________

15. Define volatile solvents.

    ____

16. As liquids evaporate, they form ______________. These can be reduced by ______________ the lids/covers of product containers.

17. A. Define *mist*.

    ____

    B. The type of mist that is difficult to control and more hazardous to breathe is a/an ______________ mist. This is produced by a/an ______________ container.

    C. Less hazardous mists are created by ______________ sprayers, and these sprayers should be used whenever possible.

18. Explain why dust masks are ineffective against vapors.

    ____

19. A. Define *odor*.

    ____

    B. Explain how odors do or do not indicate the safety of a product.

    ____

    C. List two actions of proper ventilation.

    1. ______________________________

    2. ______________________________

20. Identify two preventive steps that can be taken to avoid eating hazardous chemicals.

 1. ______________________________

 2. ______________________________

21. A. 45% of cosmetic-related injuries seen in hospital emergency rooms are to the

 ______________.

 B. In order to avoid this type of injury in question 21.A, you should wear ______________.

TOXICITY AND CARCINOGENICITY

22. A. Identify the name of the principle that determines toxicity.

 ____

 B. This principle says that toxicity is determined by the ______________ of chemical substances.

23. List three sales and marketing terms that have little, or no, true meaning.

 1. ______________________________

 2. ______________________________

 3. ______________________________

24. A chemical that causes cancer is called a/an ______________

25. List twelve rules of salon safety.

 1. ______________________________

 2. ______________________________

 3. ______________________________

 4. ______________________________

 5. ______________________________

 6. ______________________________

7. ______________________________

8. ______________________________

9. ______________________________

10. ______________________________

____

11. ______________________________

12. ______________________________

WORD REVIEW

absorption
acute effects
carcinogenic
chronic effects
dust mask
flammable
inhalation
Material Safety Data Sheets (MSDSs)
mists
nontoxic
overexposure principle
toxic
vapors
volatile
solvents

Review Test

1. The systematic study of our universe is known as:
   A. biology.
   B. science.
   C. cosmetology.
   D. anatomy. ____

2. All of the following are steps of the scientific method EXCEPT:
   A. observation.
   B. reasoning.
   C. testing.
   D. marketing. ____

3. Using information to reach a conclusion or make a decision is the power of:
   A. reasoning.
   B. testing.
   C. sales.
   D. the unknown. ____

4. Carefully evaluation of the results of the services you perform on your clients is part of:
   A. observation.
   B. testing.
   C. cause.
   D. reasoning. ____

5. A mixture that could be hazardous is known as a/an mixture.
   A. compatible
   B. miracle
   C. safe
   D. incompatible ____

6. Whose instructions should you follow when using any chemical?
   A. your instructor's
   B. the manufacturer's
   C. your co-worker's
   D. none of the above are correct ____

7. Ammonia can be deadly if it is mixed with:
   A. thioglycolic acid.
   B. aniline derivative.
   C. chlorine bleach.
   D. sodium persulfates. ____

8. All of the following are possible reactions of hazardous mixtures EXCEPT:
   A. fire.
   B. absorption.
   C. harmful vapors.
   D. explosion. ____

9. The best way to check your reasoning is by:
   A. testing.
   B. reading.
   C. following manufacturer's directions.
   D. performing predisposition tests ____

10. Keeping accurate, detailed records helps hairstylists to avoid:
    A. new procedures.
    B. changing a formula.
    C. repeating mistakes.
    D. all of the above. ____

11. The study of living things is known as:
    A. anatomy.
    B. psychology.
    C. biology.
    D. anthropology. ____

12. Plants, animals, and bacteria all contain:
    A. carbon.
    B. nitrogen.
    C. gold.
    D. hydrogen. ____

13. All of the following are made by the COHNS elements EXCEPT:
    A. blood.
    B. skin.
    C. hair.
    D. nails. ____

14. When two or more elements combine chemically, they form a/an:
    A. cell.
    B. molecule.
    C. element.
    D. compound. ____

15. Compounds that contain carbon are:
    A. inorganic.
    B. elements.
    C. organic.
    D. cytoplasm. ____

16. The control center of a cell is the:
    A. cell membrane.
    B. cytoplasm.
    C. cell wall.
    D. nucleus. _____

17. Small bodies that the nucleus uses to perform the cell's work are:
    A. organs.
    B. amino acids.
    C. keratin cells.
    D. organelles. _____

18. Cells multiply by a process of cell division that is called:
    A. keratinization.
    B. mitosis.
    C. oxidation.
    D. mitochondria. _____

19. Large, complex molecules made when amino acids bond together are:
    A. COHNS.
    B. organelles.
    C. proteins.
    D. elements. _____

20. How many types of amino acids are in the body?
    A. 5
    B. 10
    C. 15
    D. 20 _____

21. Pathogenic bacteria:
    A. may be helpful.
    B. produce disease.
    C. are harmless.
    D. none of the above are correct. _____

22. Nonpathogenic bacteria:
    A. may be helpful.
    B. produce disease.
    C. are harmless.
    D. both A and C are correct. _____

23. Bacteria cells reproduce by dividing in:
    A. half.
    B. quarters.
    C. thirds.
    D. eighths. _____

24. Bacteria are also known as germs or:
    A. viruses.
    B. fungi.
    C. microbes.
    D. verrucae. ______

25. Motility is caused by the whip-like motion of tiny, hair-like projections known as:
    A. flagella.
    B. cilia.
    C. both A and B are correct.
    D. none of the above are correct. ______

26. The inactive stage in the life cycle of bacteria is known as the:
    A. pathogenic stage.
    B. spore-forming stage.
    C. infection stage.
    D. nonpathogenic state. ______

27. Viruses:
    A. are smaller than bacteria.
    B. do not have a cell structure.
    C. can't live outside the body.
    D. A, B, and C are all correct. ______

28. The HIV virus causes:
    A. AIDS.
    B. influenza.
    C. herpes.
    D. none of the above are correct. ______

29. HIV is easily killed by:
    A. alcohol.
    B. chlorine bleach.
    C. both A and B are correct.
    D. none of the above are correct. ______

30. Acquired immunity is a resistance to disease that occurs:
    A. as a result of inoculation.
    B. after the body overcomes a disease.
    C. both A and B are correct.
    D. none of the above are correct. ______

31. The type of tissue that gives a protective covering to the body is:
    A. epithelial.
    B. liquid.
    C. connective.
    D. muscular. ______

32. All of the following are layers of the skin EXCEPT:
    A. dermis.
    B. subcutaneous tissue.
    C. epidermis.
    D. cortex. _____

33. The substance in the skin that gives it strength and is also used to make glue is:
    A. elastin.
    B. keratin.
    C. collagen.
    D. melanin. _____

34. The skin's cells that release a chemical to stop bleeding are known as _____________________ cells.
    A. viral
    B. elastin
    C. stratum
    D. mast _____

35. The type of tissue that carries instructions from the brain to other body parts is:
    A. muscular.
    B. nerve.
    C. connective.
    D. epithelial. _____

36. The substance in the skin that gives it stretchability is:
    A. lymph.
    B. adipose tissue.
    C. collagen.
    D. elastin. _____

37. The largest organ of the body is the:
    A. skin.
    B. heart.
    C. lungs.
    D. liver. _____

38. The outermost layer of the skin is the:
    A. adipose tissue.
    B. epidermis.
    C. subcutaneous tissue.
    D. dermis. _____

39. The name of the gland that secretes sebum is:
    A. suderiferous.
    B. arrector pili.
    C. sebaceous.
    D. pituitary. _____

40. The name of the skin's pigment is:
 A. keratin.
 B. melanin.
 C. elastin.
 D. sebum. _____

41. How much sebum does the body make every 100 days?
 A. 1 ounce
 B. 1 pint
 C. 1 quart
 D. 1 gallon _____

42 The name of the muscle that causes goosebumps is:
 A. sebaceous.
 B. papilla.
 C. arrector pili.
 D. suderiferous. _____

43. The innermost portion of the hair shaft is the:
 A. cortex.
 B. medulla.
 C. collagen.
 D. cuticle. _____

44. The layer of the hair that makes up 90% of its total weight is the:
 A. cortex.
 B. epidermis.
 C. cuticle.
 D. medulla. _____

45. Long, coiled chains of amino acids are known as:
 A. cystine.
 B. cysteine.
 C. helix.
 D. polypeptides. _____

46. Side bonds that occur between two sulfur atoms are:
 A. simple proteins.
 B. polypeptides.
 C. capillaries.
 D. disulfide bonds. _____

47. The most abundant amino acid in the hair is:
 A. keratin.
 B. sebum.
 C. cystine.
 D. melanin. _____

48. At least nine fiber chains twisted to make a larger bundle are known as:
   A. micro fibrils.
   B. amino acids.
   C. macro fibrils.
   D. cystine. _____

49. In which hair layer is the coloring pigment found?
   A. medulla
   B. cortex
   C. cuticle
   D. none of the above are correct _____

50. Which hair layer has cells that overlap like roof shingles?
   A. medulla
   B. dermis
   C. cuticle
   D. cortex _____

51. The name of the hair's growth phase/cycle is:
   A. telogen.
   B. keratinization.
   C. catagen.
   D. anagen. _____

52. All of the following are characteristics of vellus hair EXCEPT that it is:
   A. coarse.
   B. short.
   C. soft.
   D. fine. _____

53. All of the following are types of secondary terminal hair EXCEPT hair on the:
   A. scalp.
   B. eyelashes.
   C. back.
   D. legs. _____

54. When the hair's bulb separates from the papilla and lies loosely in the follicle, the hair is known as:
   A. elliptical.
   B. anagen.
   C. bed-hair.
   D. shed-hair. _____

55. The type of melanin that gives hair yellowish-blond tones is:
   A. para-melanin.
   B. phaeomelanin.
   C. eumalanin.
   D. melanocytes _____

56. The number of hairs growing in a square inch of scalp is known as the hair's:
 A. elasticity.
 B. texture.
 C. density.
 D. porosity. _____

57. The phase/cycle when the hair is resting is called:
 A. telogen.
 B. catagen.
 C. anagen.
 D. both A and C are correct. _____

58. All of the following are classifications of hair diameter EXCEPT:
 A. thick.
 B. coarse.
 C. medium.
 D. fine. _____

59. The vitamin that appears to cause hair loss is vitamin:
 A. A
 B. B
 C. D
 D. E _____

60. The structural strength, volume, and resiliency of hair is known as hair:
 A. texture.
 B. porosity.
 C. elasticity.
 D. body. _____

61. Anything that occupies space and has mass is:
 A. energy.
 B. carbon.
 C. matter.
 D. bacteria. _____

62. Which of the following can flow and take the shape of their container?
 A. solids
 B. elements
 C. liquids
 D. both A and C are correct _____

63. The simplest form of matter is a/an:
 A. element.
 B. compound.
 C. chemical.
 D. solution. _____

64. All of the following are examples of natural polymers EXCEPT:
    A. wood.
    B. silk.
    C. leather.
    D. epoxy. ____

65. Any substance capable of dissolving another substance is a/an:
    A. solute.
    B. solvent.
    C. emulsion.
    D. insoluble. ____

66. The most energetic wavelength is a ____________________ wavelength.
    A. long
    B. medium
    C. short
    D. none of the above are correct ____

67. A white object stays cool in temperature because it ____________________ all wavelengths of visible light.
    A. absorbs
    B. reflects
    C. accepts
    D. none of the above are correct ____

68. What type of change is a change of state?
    A. a chemical change
    B. a physical change
    C. a volatile change
    D. none of the above are correct ____

69. What type of change occurs when matter changes its chemical structure?
    A. physical
    B. emotional
    C. mental
    D. chemical ____

70. The smallest particle of an element that still behaves like an element is a/an:
    A. compound.
    B. atom.
    C. polymer.
    D. emulsion. ____

71. Another name for alkaline is:
    A. acid.
    B. pH.
    C. neutral.
    D. basic. ____

72. A product that has a pH level of 4.5 is:
    A. acidic.
    B. neutral.
    C. alkaline.
    D. none of the above are correct. ____

73. Moisture in the skin and scalp combined with sebum is known as:
    A. pH balanced.
    B. acid mantle.
    C. neutralized.
    D. acid-balanced. ____

74. Any chemical, acid or alkaline, that is capable of rapidly destroying human tissue is known as a/an:
    A. balancer.
    B. emulsifier
    C. corrosive.
    D. neutralizer. ____

75. All of the following cosmetology services depend on oxidizing agents EXCEPT:
    A. permanent waving.
    B. hair lightening.
    C. haircoloring.
    D. hydroxide relaxers. ____

76. All of the following are examples of oxidizing agents EXCEPT:
    A. peroxides.
    B. bromates.
    C. persulfates.
    D. chlorine bleach. ____

77. An example of a reducing agent is:
    A. ammonium thioglycolate.
    B. hydrogen peroxide.
    C. perborate.
    D. sodium bromate. ____

78. A substance that dissolves in oil is:
    A. hydrophilic.
    B. a detergent.
    C. lipophilic.
    D. an insoluble solution. ____

79. A solution that has a pH level of 13 is a/an:
    A. acid.
    B. neutral product.
    C. alkaline.
    D. pH-balanced product. ____

80. All of the following are safety precautions to be taken when using reducing agents EXCEPT:
    A. wear gloves.
    B. wear eye protection.
    C. store with oxidizers.
    D. use proper ventilation. ____

81. Which of the following are chemicals?
    A. pure water
    B. ammonia
    C. oxygen
    D. all of the above ____

82. The principle that deals with safe and unsafe levels of chemical exposure is known as the

    ____________________ principle.
    A. overexposure
    B. chemical reaction
    C. folklore
    D. carcinogenic ____

83. The Occupational Safety and Health Administration is part of the ____________________ government.
    A. city
    B. local
    C. state
    D. federal ____

84. A Material Safety Data Sheet gives all of the following information about a product EXCEPT:
    A. safe handling techniques.
    B. emergency first aid advice.
    C. potentially hazardous ingredients found in each product.
    D. that employers are required to provide a safe working environment. ____

85. All of the following will adversely affect many products EXCEPT:
    A. extreme cold.
    B. darkness.
    C. excessive heat.
    D. light. ____

86. Overexposure effects for long periods of time are known as ____________________ effects.
    A. acute
    B. MSDS
    C. chronic
    D. entry ____

87. Solvents that evaporate quickly are called:
    A. mists.
    B. toxic.
    C. volatile.
    D. flammable. ____

88. A chemical that causes cancer is a/an:
   A. vapor.
   B. carcinogen.
   C. HIV virus.
   D. chemophobia. ____

89. All of the following are the body's routes of entry EXCEPT:
   A. unbroken skin.
   B. inhalation.
   C. broken skin.
   D. ingestion. ____

90. The Employee Right to Know Act is a regulation of:
   A. MSDS.
   B. state cosmetology agencies.
   C. FDA.
   D. OSHA. ____

91. The person who should treat irritant contact dermatitis is a:
   A. cosmetologist.
   B. manicurist/nail technician.
   C. dermatologist.
   D. dentist. ____

92. An allergic reaction that occurs when a person becomes sensitized to a product ingredient is called:
   A. allergic contact dermatitis.
   B. pityriasis.
   C. irritant contact dermatitis.
   D. alopecia. ____

93. Another name for sensitizer is:
   A. allergen.
   B. preservative.
   C. aniline derivative.
   D. irritant. ____

94. An advanced form of allergic dermatitis is:
   A. pediculosis.
   B. chronic eczema.
   C. alopecia areata.
   D. hypertrichosis. ____

95. A common sensitizer is:
   A. tap water.
   B. sodium laurel sulfate.
   C. formaldehyde.
   D. sodium laureth sulfate. ____

96. The metal that is one of the most common allergens in the world is:
    A. gold.
    B. lead.
    C. silver.
    D. nickel. ____

97. Disposable gloves are made out of the following materials:
    A. PVA.
    B. nitrile.
    C. latex.
    D. both B and C are correct. ____

98. The number one occupation-related disease in the United States is ______________________ disease.
    A. heart
    B. skin
    C. lung
    D. AIDS ____

99. Irritant contact dermatitis can chemically damage the epidermis and the:
    A. dermis.
    B. subcutaneous tissue.
    C. cortex.
    D. adipose tissue. ____

100. The process of prolonged or repeated contact with an allergen is called:
    A. allergic reaction.
    B. sensitization.
    C. eczema.
    D. irritant contact dermatitis. ____

101. Soap is a type of:
    A. preservative.
    B. emulsifier.
    C. disinfectant.
    D. detergent. ____

102. All of the following are oils used in making soap EXCEPT:
    A. sebum.
    B. palm.
    C. olive.
    D. castor. ____

103. A surface active agent is also called a/an:
    A. detergent.
    B. conditioner.
    C. emulsifier.
    D. surfactant. ____

104. Antibacterial surfactants with a positive charge are:
A. negative ions.
B. amphoteric.
C. positive ions.
D. cationic.
____

105. A surfactant with a negative charge is:
A. saponin.
B. nonionic.
C. cationic.
D. anionic.
____

106. A substance that prevents film from depositing on the hair shaft is a/an:
A. opacifier.
B. chelator.
C. pearling agent.
D. thickener.
____

107. An ingredient that inhibits bacteria growth is a/an:
A. surfactant.
B. foam builder.
C. preservative.
D. opacifier.
____

108. Another name for overactive sebaceous glands is:
A. seborrhea.
B. suderiferous.
C. pityriasis capitis simplex.
D. pediculosis.
____

109. A substance that attracts moisture to the skin and scalp is a:
A. fatty material.
B. protein derivative.
C. humectant.
D. lanolin-based moisturizer.
____

110. What are the most common volatile organic compounds used in hairspray?
A. SD alcohols
B. alkanolamines
C. chlorofluorocarbons
D. all of the above are correct
____

111. Red, blue, and yellow are ______________________ colors.
A. primary
B. secondary
C. tertiary
D. quaternary
____

112. The balance of color indicates its:
   A. depth.
   B. lightness.
   C. tone.
   D. darkness. ____

113. Two colors opposite each other on the color wheel are ____________________ colors.
   A. primary
   B. quaternary
   C. saturation
   D. complementary ____

114. The type of melanin that gives hair shades from brown to black is:
   A. keratin.
   B. sebum.
   C. eumelanin.
   D. phaeomelanin. ____

115. The process of melanin being altered so that it no longer absorbs visible light is called:
   A. decolorization.
   B. haircoloring.
   C. depositing.
   D. neutralization. ____

116. The degree of concentration or pigment in a color is:
   A. tone.
   B. value.
   C. saturation.
   D. complementary. ____

117. A chemical used to make the pH level of peroxide alkaline is:
   A. citric acid.
   B. ammonia.
   C. thioglycolic acid.
   D. chlorine bleach. ____

118. All of the following parts of the hair are affected by oxidation EXCEPT:
   A. medulla.
   B. keratin.
   C. melanin.
   D. disulfide bonds. ____

119. The pH level of stabilized hydrogen peroxide is:
   A. below 4.
   B. 7.
   C. 9.
   D. 14. ____

120. A noticeable increase in porosity from the scalp to the hair ends is called porosity ____________________:
A. control.
B. gradients.
C. stretch.
D. building. ____

121. Nonoxidation haircolors:
A. are not mixed with developer or activator.
B. deposit color without lightening the natural color.
C. both A and B are correct.
D. none of the above are correct. ____

122. Haircolors that deposit color without lightening the natural hair color are:
A. semi-permanent colors.
B. demi-permanent colors.
C. both A and B are correct.
D. none of the above are correct ____

123. The amount of lift in permanent haircolors is controlled by the:
A. pH
B. concentration of peroxide
C. ammonia
D. both A and B are correct. ____

124. Processing a haircolor service at 90°F instead of 72°F will cause the color to:
A. fade less.
B. process twice as fast.
C. be a lighter color.
D. A, B, and C are all correct. ____

125. A substance that colors prelightened hair to a delicate shade is a:
A. dye solvent.
B. haircolor.
C. chelator.
D. toner. ____

126. A product that penetrates broken cuticles and fills small holes in the hair is a/an:
A. developer.
B. enzyme activator.
C. primary intermediate.
D. filler. ____

127. The application of an oxidizing haircolor to hair that has been previously colored with metallic dyes may:
A. melt and destroy the hair.
B. cause the color to be lighter.
C. cause the color to be darker.
D. cause an unwanted shade. ____

128. Lead, copper, and silver are examples of:
A. henna.
B. metallic dyes.
C. tertiary colors.
D. vegetable dyes. ____

129. To determine if a client is allergic to a product, a ____________________ test should be performed.
A. match
B. predisposition
C. elasticity
D. strand ____

130. A substance that damages genetic material and affects future generations is a:
A. mutagen.
B. teratogen.
C. carcinogen.
D. none of the above. ____

131. Amino acids are linked together, end-to-end, by ____________________ bonds.
A. peptide
B. disulfide
C. ionic
D. hydrogen ____

132. Wetting the hair breaks the ____________________ bonds.
A. peptide
B. disulfide
C. ionic
D. hydrogen ____

133. The reducing agent that is only found in acid-balanced perms is:
A. sodium bromate.
B. glyceryl monothioglycolate.
C. hydrogen peroxide.
D. none of the above. ____

134. The most widely used reducer in alkaline perms is:
A. sodium persulfate.
B. hydrogen peroxide.
C. ammonium thioglycolate.
D. monothioglycolate. ____

135. The hair's ability to absorb liquids is called its:
A. density.
B. elasticity.
C. porosity.
D. texture. ____

136. The hair's cortex layer is made up of millions of amino acid chains known as:
A. organelles.
B. polypeptides.
C. keratinizations.
D. polymers. _____

137. Salt bonds are a type of ____________________ bond.
A. peptide
B. hydrogen
C. disulfide
D. ionic _____

138. The bond that is broken during permanent waving is a/an:
A. disulfide bond.
B. peptide bond.
C. end bond.
D. polypeptide bond. _____

139. Another name for a self-heating perm is:
A. endothermic.
B. exothermic.
C. acid-balanced perm.
D. fixative. _____

140. An oxidizer found in most neutralizers is:
A. sodium hydroxide.
B. thioglycolate.
C. aniline derivative.
D. hydrogen peroxide. _____

141. Hair that has a smaller diameter than normal/average hair is known as ____________________ hair.
A. coarse
B. resistant
C. medium
D. fine _____

142. When the many side bonds normally found in hair are temporarily broken, the hair is said to be in a/an ____________________ state.
A. expanded
B. resistant
C. reduced
D. growth _____

143. In chemical relaxing, combing and pulling on the hair are known as ____________________ actions.
A. chemical
B. physical
C. biological
D. metaphysical _____

144. The thickness of a product refers to its:
   A. viscosity.
   B. porosity.
   C. abundance.
   D. strength. ____

145. All of the following terms refer to the same thing EXCEPT:
   A. hydrogen peroxide.
   B. sodium hydroxide.
   C. lye.
   D. caustic soda. ____

146. All of the following are alkaline relaxers EXCEPT:
   A. potassium hydroxide.
   B. lithium hydroxide.
   C. guanidine hydroxide.
   D. aniline derivative. ____

147. A petroleum cream designed to protect the scalp from damage is a:
   A. depilatory cream.
   B. cleansing cream.
   C. base cream.
   D. none of the above. ____

148. The hair's ability to stretch and return to its original length without breaking is known as its:
   A. porosity.
   B. elasticity.
   C. density.
   D. texture. ____

149. The neutralizer used in hydroxide relaxers:
   A. rebuilds disulfide bonds by oxidation.
   B. rebuilds disulfide bonds by lanthionization.
   C. neutralizes alkaline residues with an acidic pH.
   D. rebuilds disulfide bonds by reduction. ____

150. Hair that has been previously relaxed with a thio relaxer should not be treated with a/an

   ____________________ relaxer.
   A. aniline
   B. sodium perborate
   C. hydroxide
   D. thio ____

Notes

Notes

Notes

Notes

Notes

Notes

Notes

Notes

Notes

Notes

Notes

Notes

Notes

Notes

CPSIA information can be obtained
at www.ICGtesting.com
Printed in the USA
FFOW01n1549150718
47420255-50648FF

9 781428 335615